The Plant Pledge

by: Kate Murray

illustrated by:

Sarah Geraci

foreward by:

Aparna Mele, MD

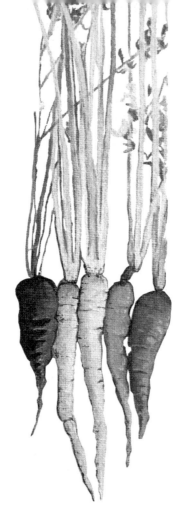

$19.99
ISBN 978-0-9859972-3-6
51999>

9 780985 997236

For Carla & Joe,
thank you for being my inspiration.
May you have the courage
to lead a life of happiness and balance.
And always remember
eating fruit on a kabob.

For Steve,
thank you for continuing to eat
strange plants that you've never heard of.
I am forever grateful for your love and support.

KM

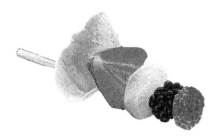

Foreward

Eating is a fundamental part of the human experience. Eating is communal; it is celebratory, sustaining, and nourishing. But in our busy and tumultuous lives, eating can become an afterthought, and turn into an emotional fix or a quick reward for the taste buds and often, we tend to lose sight of what we are eating, how we are eating it, and how it affects our bodies. I see the consequences of this daily in my practice as a gastroenterologist, where patients suffer from a host of digestive diseases directly linked to bad diets.

When I started my nonprofit organization, My Gut Instinct Inc., to educate the community about the importance of digestive health, and to inspire and compel people to eat and live better, I had the privilege of meeting and befriending Kate Murray, who became an instrumental member of my organizational team, and together we created a unique and large scale public educational health expo that succeeded in making a positive impact in our local community and beyond. From personal experience, I can attest to Kate's zealous passion of advocating for wellness through nutritional education.

According to the surgeon general, obesity today is an epidemic; it is arguably the most pressing public health problem we face, costing the health care system an estimated $90 billion a year. Three out of five Americans are overweight; one out of five is obese. Obesity is the 2nd leading preventable cause of death, behind smoking. Research has shown that plant-based diets are both cost effective and medically effective, proven to lower body mass index, blood pressure, blood sugar, and cholesterol levels. A plant-based diet can lower death rates from obesity-linked heart disease.

As a nutritional doctor and a mother myself, I found this book to be beautifully written, perfectly capturing the message of nutritional wellness and disease prevention. The message is really quite simple; adults eat the food they enjoyed as children, and children eat what you put in front of them. So, parents, simply by choosing to serve healthy fruits and vegetables to feed your family, you have the powerful ability to instill a lifetime of good dietary habits that can promote health and longevity.

I am honored to invite you to make this book part of your life. Your health and the health of your children are worth it!

Aparna Mele, M.D.
Gastroenterologist
President of My Gut Instinct, Inc.
Wyomissing, PA

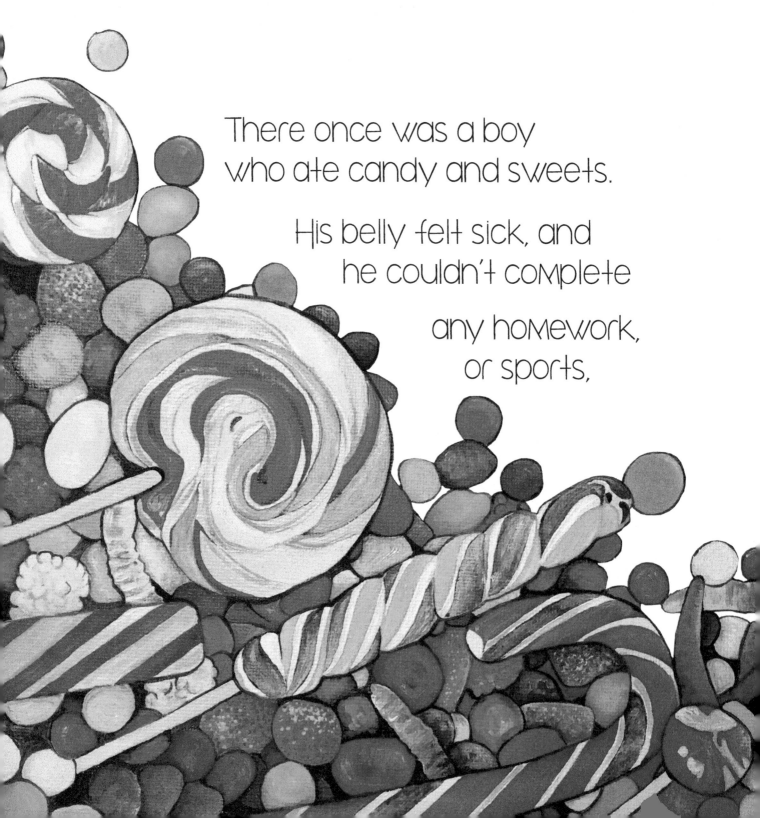

There once was a boy
who ate candy and sweets.

His belly felt sick, and
he couldn't complete

any homework,
or sports,

Music, or anything fun.

He was tired, and achy,
and grumpy and done.

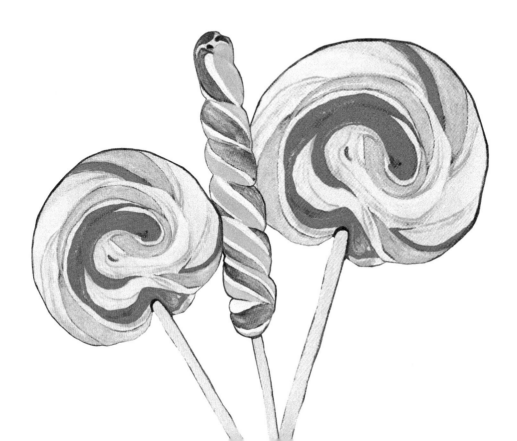

Why doesn't he feel well?
Why can't he come play?

The neighborhood
friends
and his sister
would say.

He's stuck in bed,
with an achy head,
he wants to play
but can't even
get dressed.

His mother feels sad
and overly stressed.

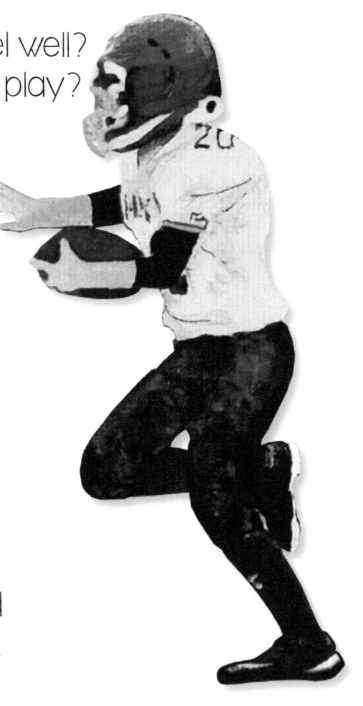

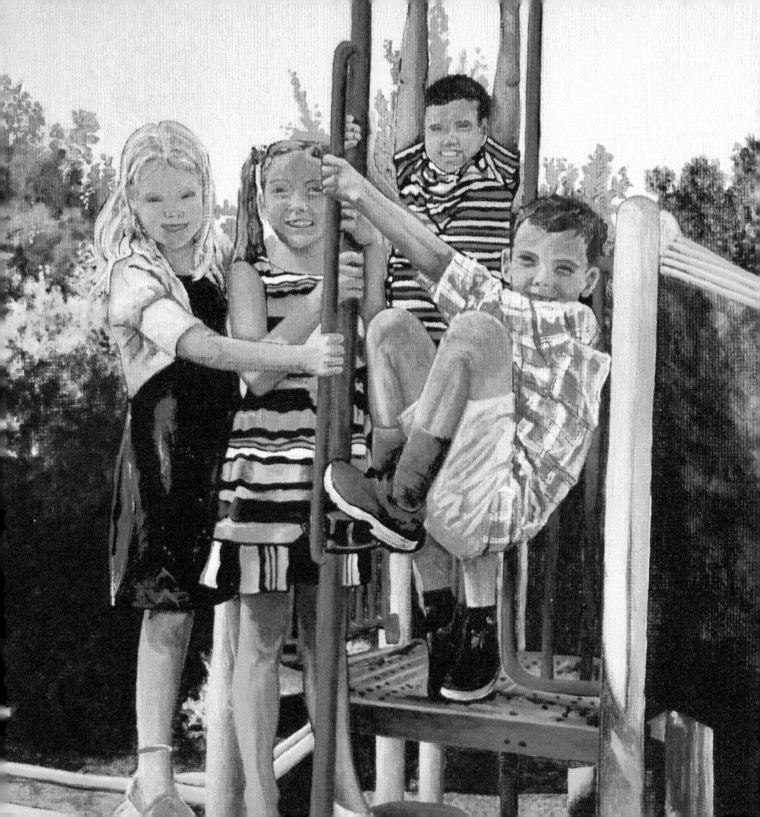

I have a secret
I'd like to share,
with you my friend,
because I care.

Eat whole foods
that grow
in the ground,
in your town,
in your yard,
in your neighbor's
mom's garden.

The ones that you know
have been treated with love,
with water and sunlight
from the sky above.

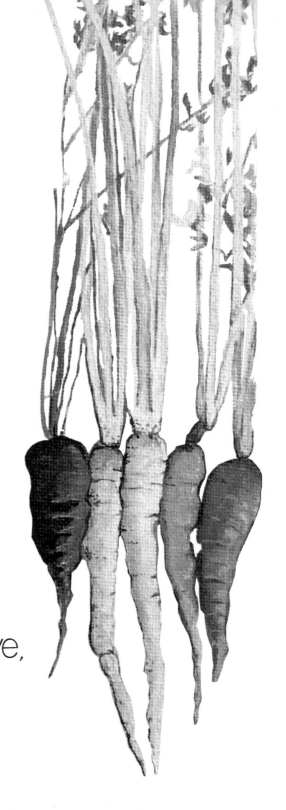

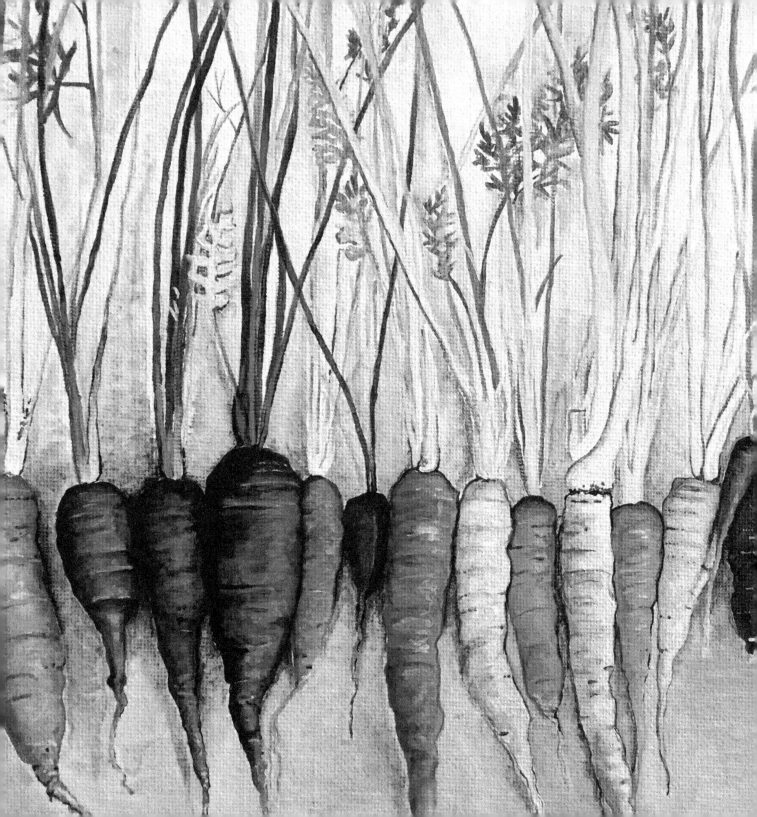

When you eat
what you grow
in your garden yourself,
your body feels good
from your nose to your toes.

You will grow up strong,
both inside and out.
Instead of a belly ache,
you can run, jump and shout!

You can kick, you can throw,
you can ski in the snow.
You can dance, you can sing,
you can splash, you can swing;
taking the pledge helps
you do all these things.

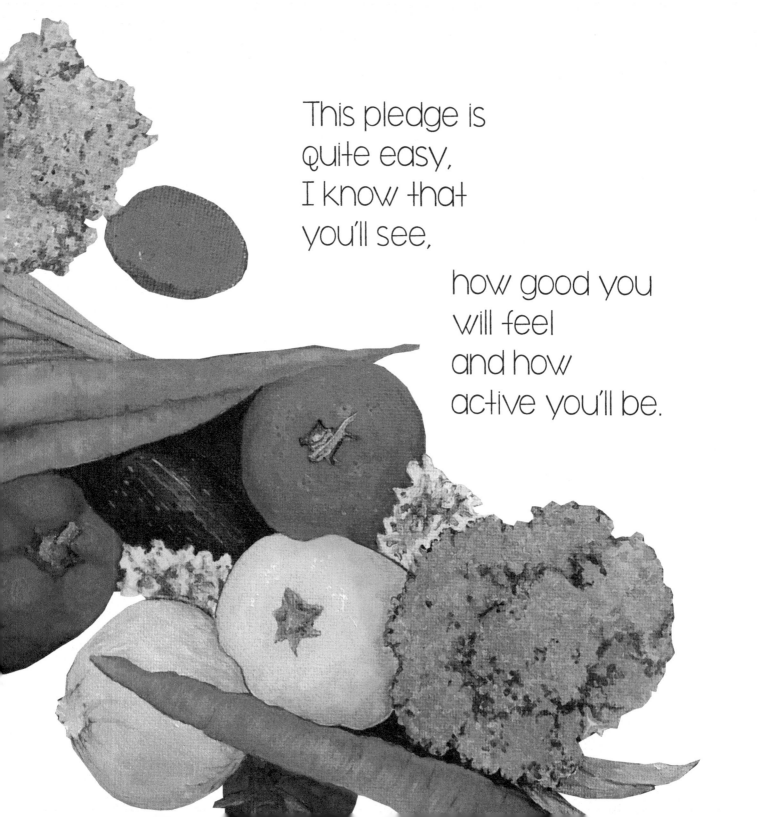

This pledge is
quite easy,
I know that
you'll see,

how good you
will feel
and how
active you'll be.

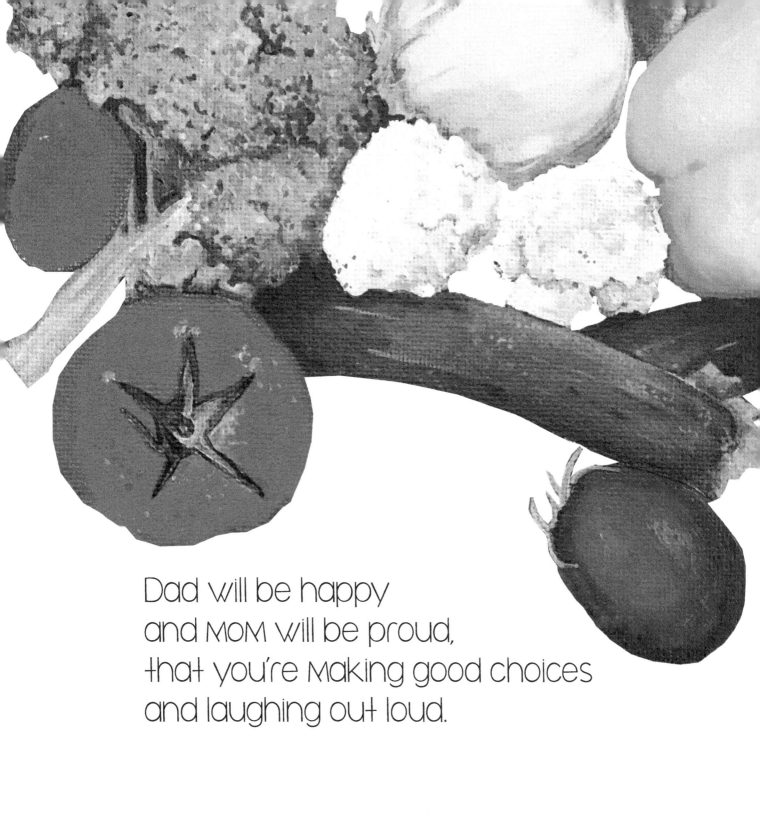

Dad will be happy
and MOM will be proud,
that you're Making good choices
and laughing out loud.

It's no secret,
these foods give you
superhero powers for days!

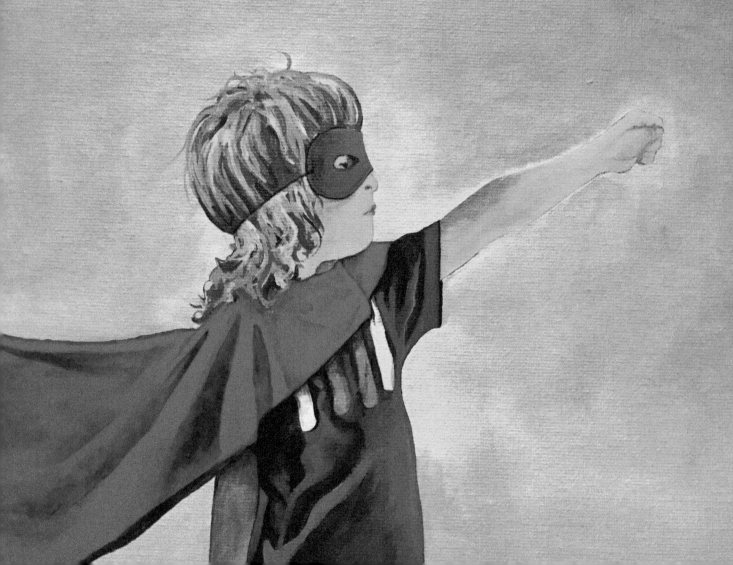

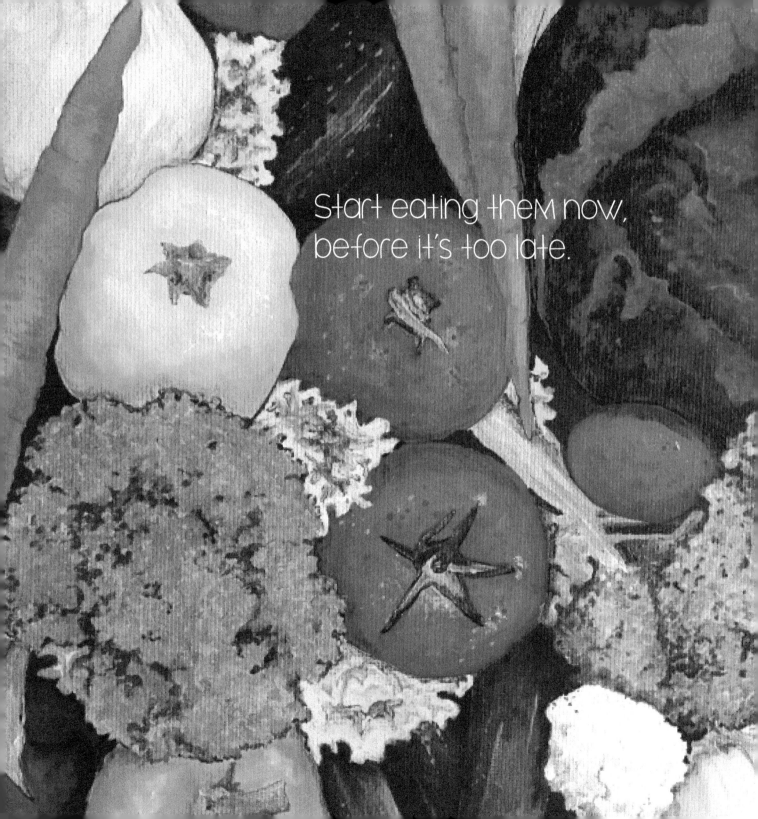

Start eating them now,
before it's too late.

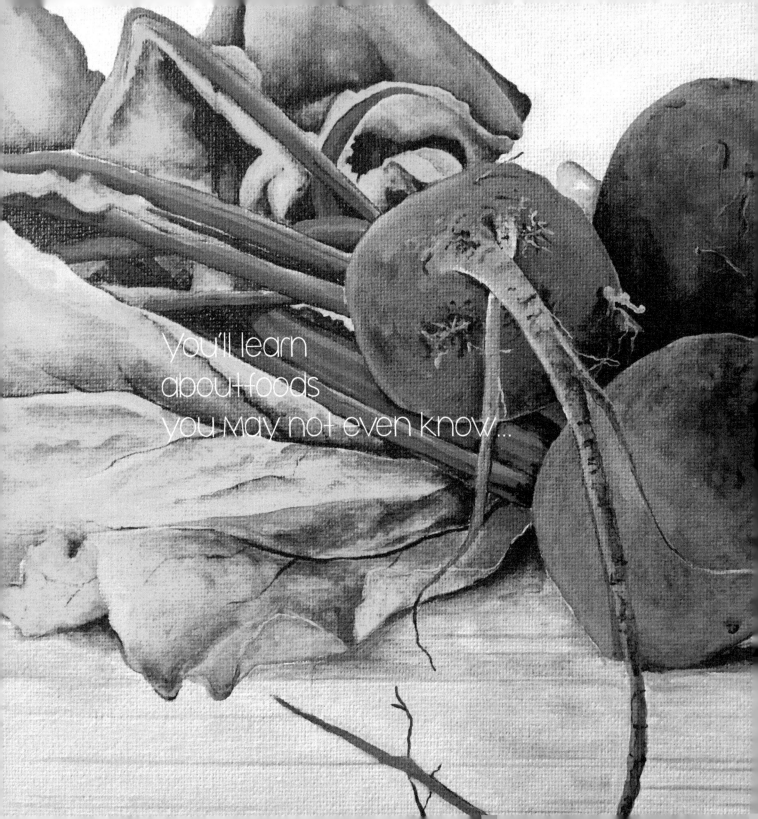

You'll learn
about foods
you may not even know...

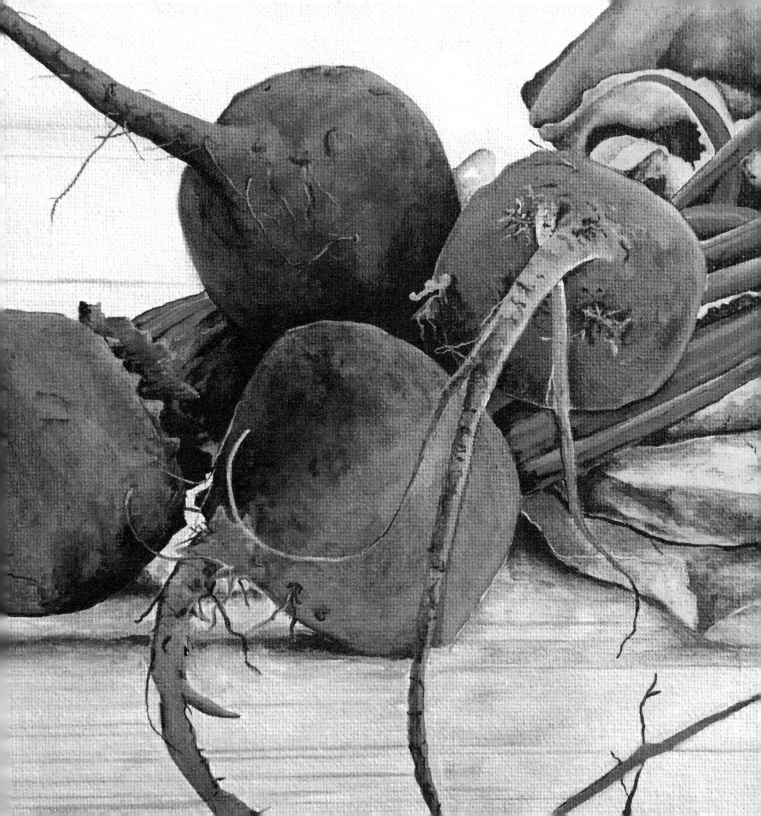

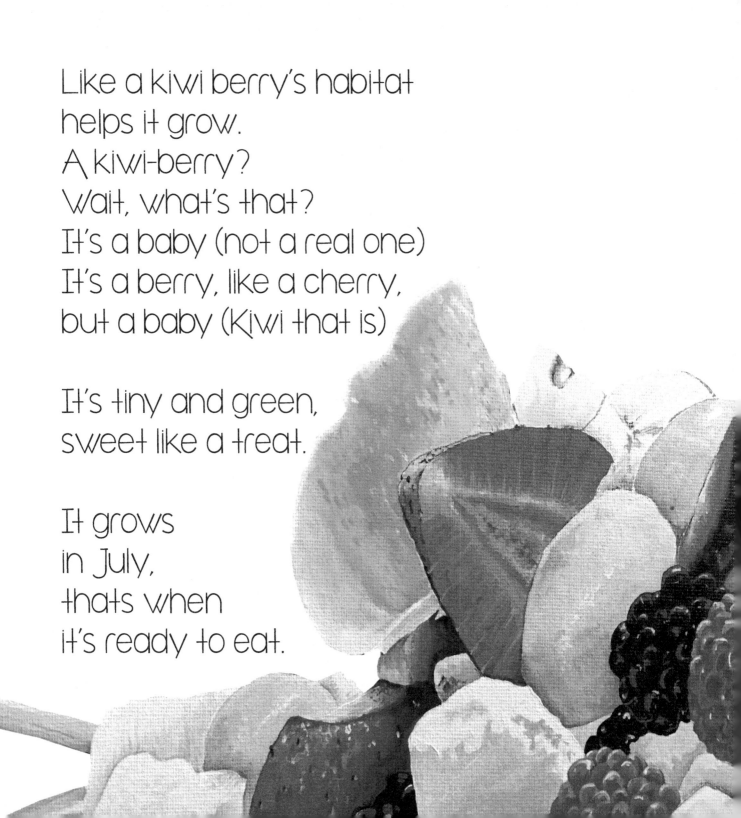

Like a kiwi berry's habitat
helps it grow.
A kiwi-berry?
Wait, what's that?
It's a baby (not a real one)
It's a berry, like a cherry,
but a baby (Kiwi that is)

It's tiny and green,
sweet like a treat.

It grows
in July,
thats when
it's ready to eat.

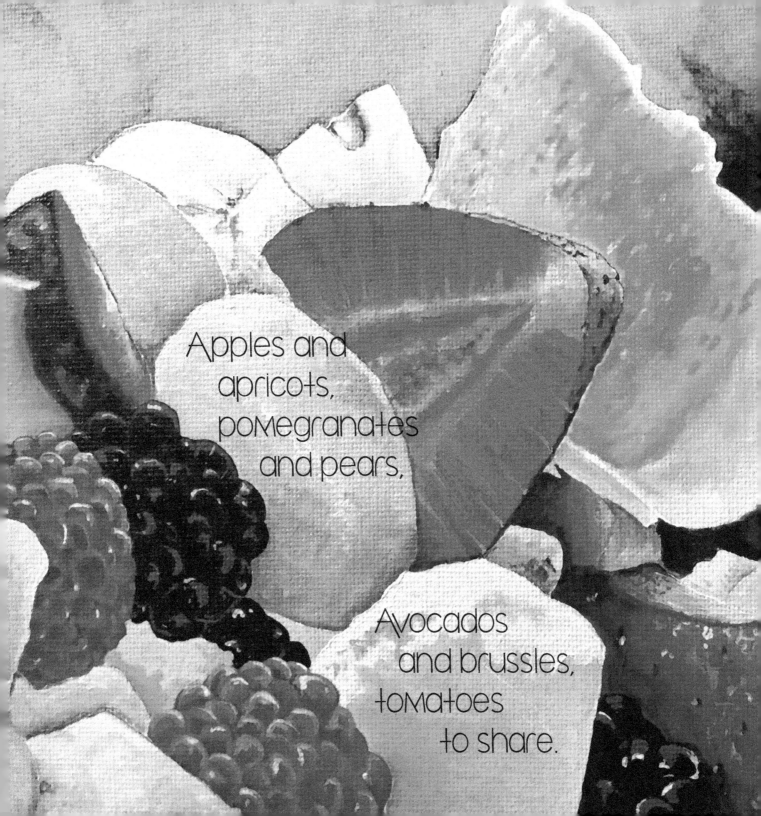

Apples and
apricots,
pomegranates
and pears,

Avocados
and brussles,
tomatoes
to share.

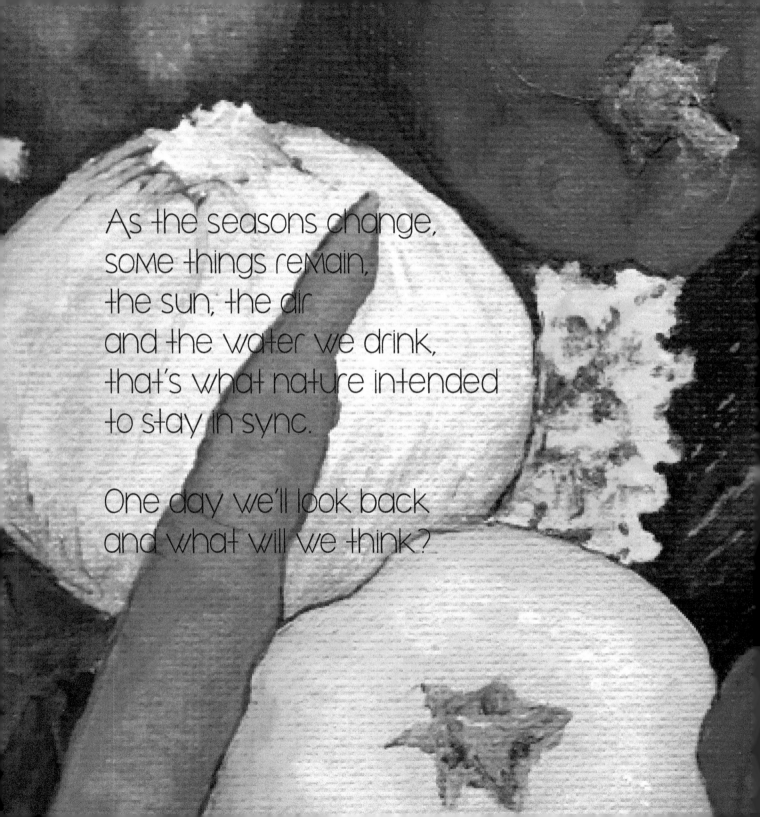

As the seasons change,
some things remain,
the sun, the air
and the water we drink,
that's what nature intended
to stay in sync.

One day we'll look back
and what will we think?

If we don't all take part
and make the change now,
Our food will keep
making us sicker,
but how?

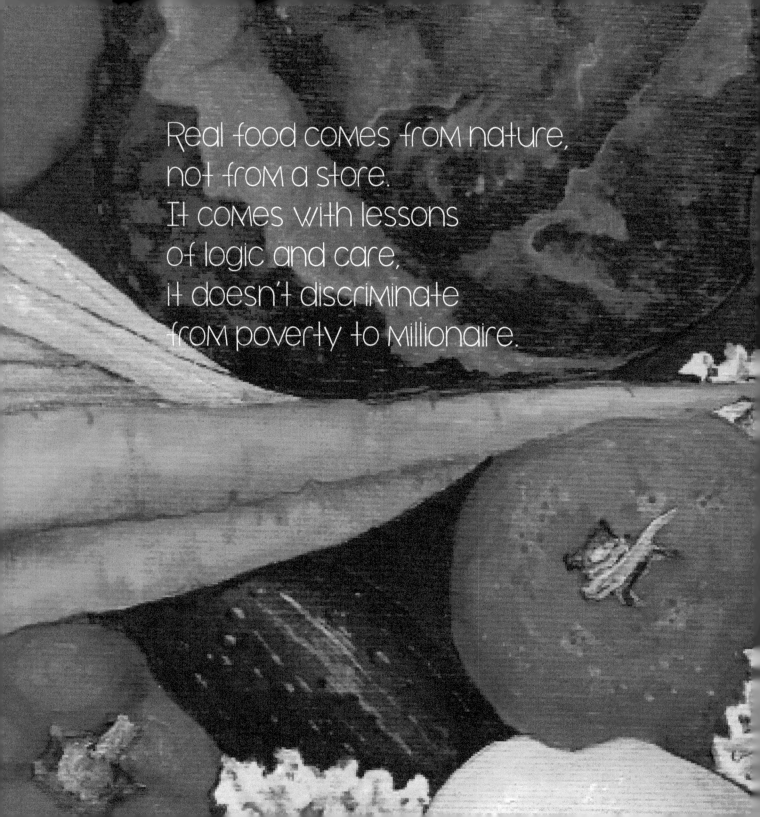

Real food comes from nature,
not from a store.
It comes with lessons
of logic and care,
It doesn't discriminate
from poverty to Millionaire.

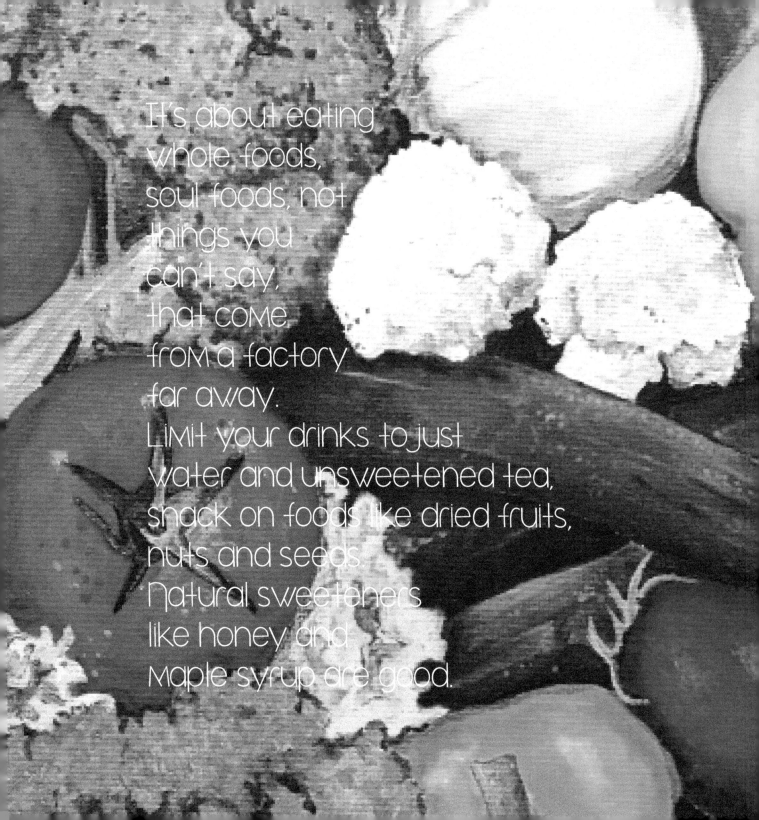

It's about eating
whole foods,
soul foods, not
things you
can't say,
that come
from a factory
far away.
Limit your drinks to just
water and unsweetened tea,
snack on foods like dried fruits,
nuts and seeds.
Natural sweeteners
like honey and
maple syrup are good.

Stay away
from packages,
boxes and
bottles too;
they contain
artificial ingredients
that you can't
pronounce,
That means
they are harmful,
even an ounce.

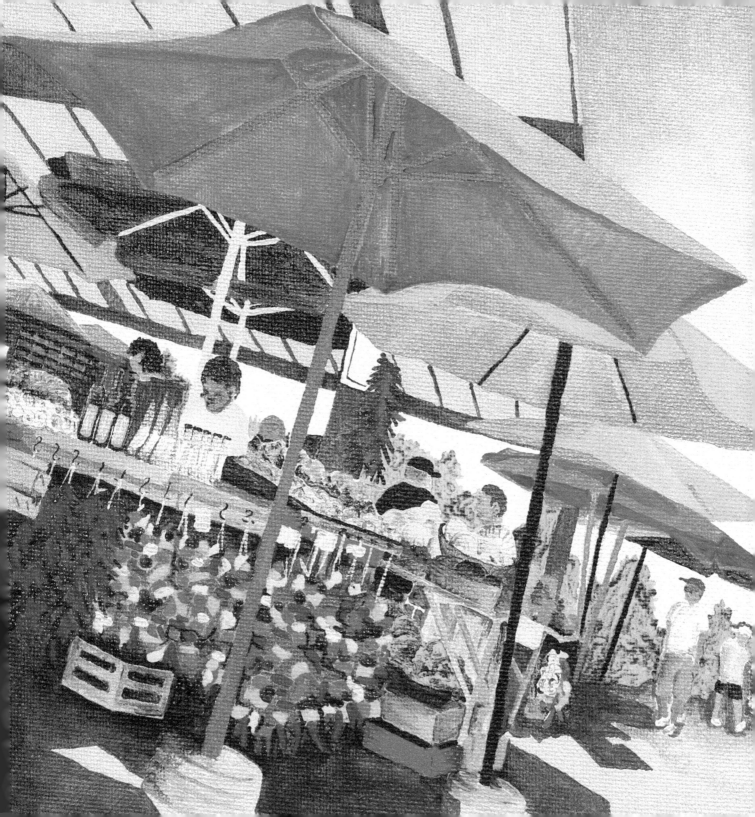

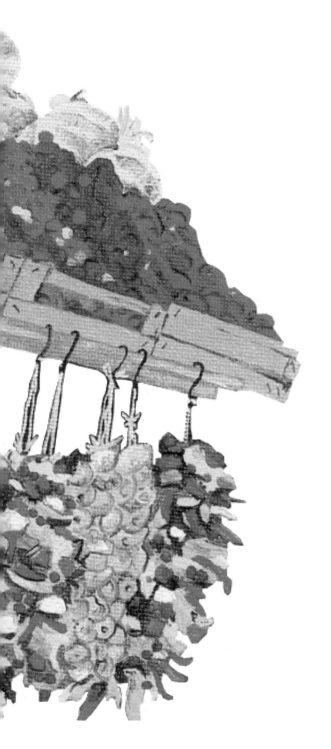

The Plant Pledge
frowns highly
upon these
"non" foods
assembled in
a faraway town.

Eat only the ones
you know
have been
treated with love,
with water
and sunlight
from the sky above.

Fruits and vegetables
nuts and seeds
Eat them every day
to prevent disease.

Eat them for breakfast,
eat them for lunch,
munch on raw veggies
for extra crunch.

Take the pledge,
I know you will.
It will do you good
and help instill
values and morals
and responsibility.

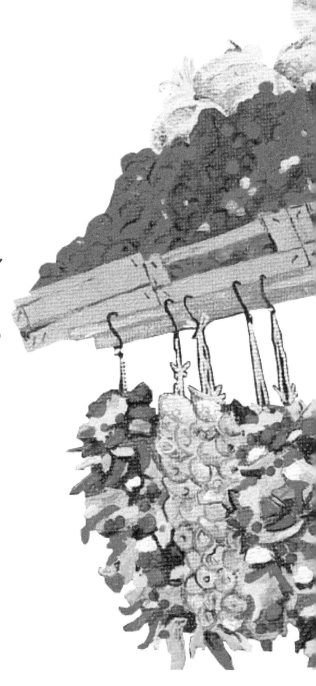

Anything red, anything green;
The brighter the color
the smarter you'll be.
It will pay off tenfold
I'll show you, come see.

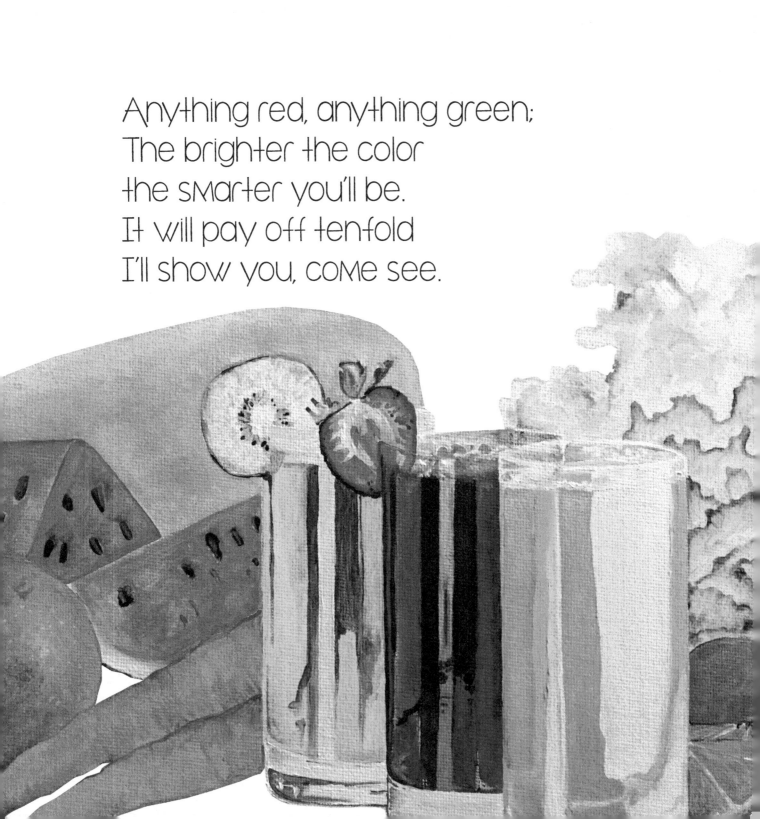

No more coughing,
or aching, or
feeling gloomy.

Chop them
or juice them,
eat the skin;
however
you like them,
just begin!

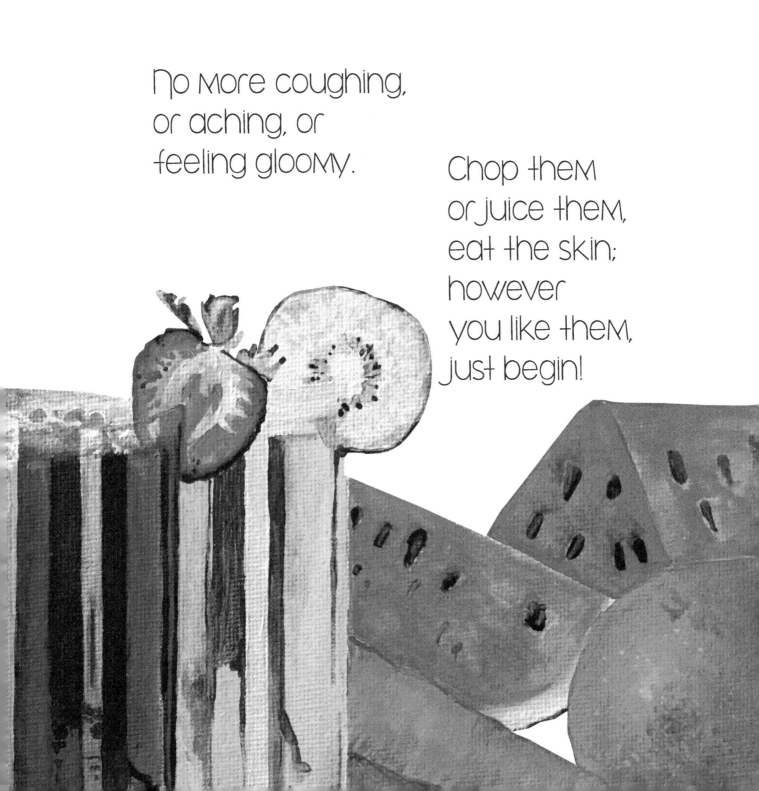

Begin today,
don't wait
until later.

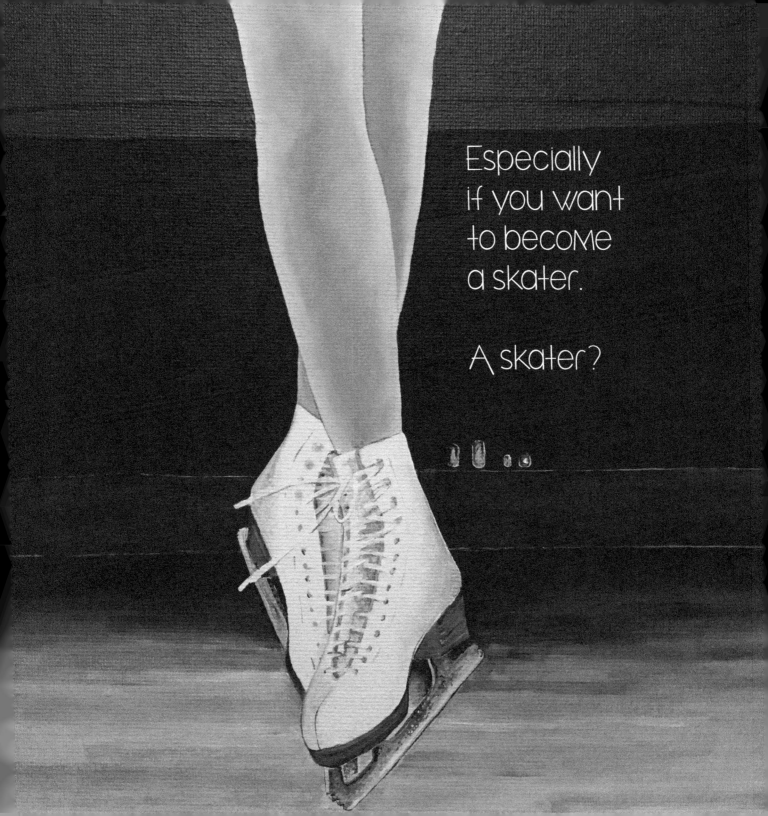

Especially
if you want
to become
a skater.

A skater?

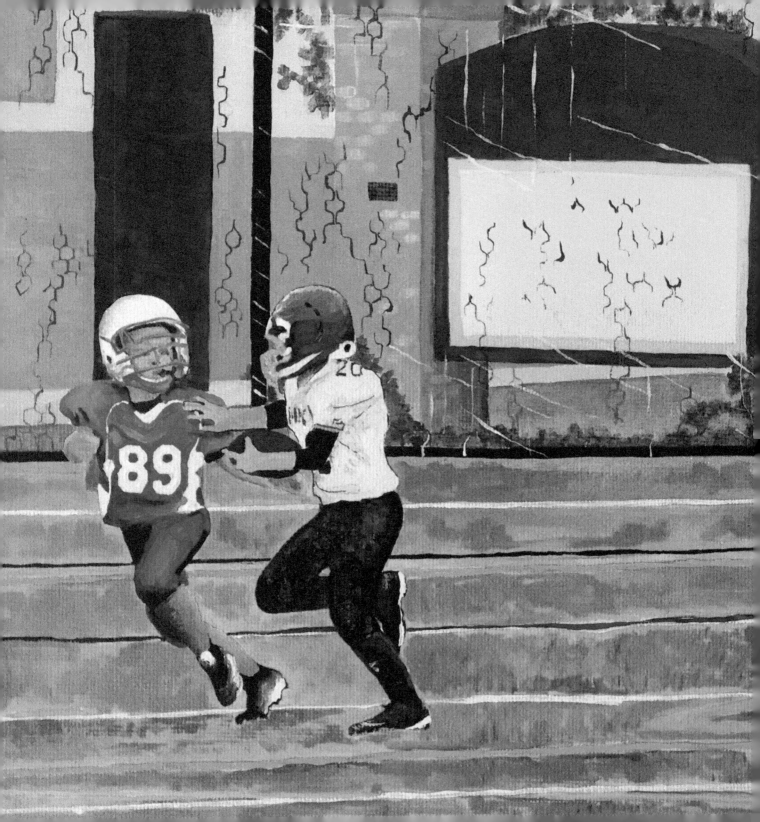

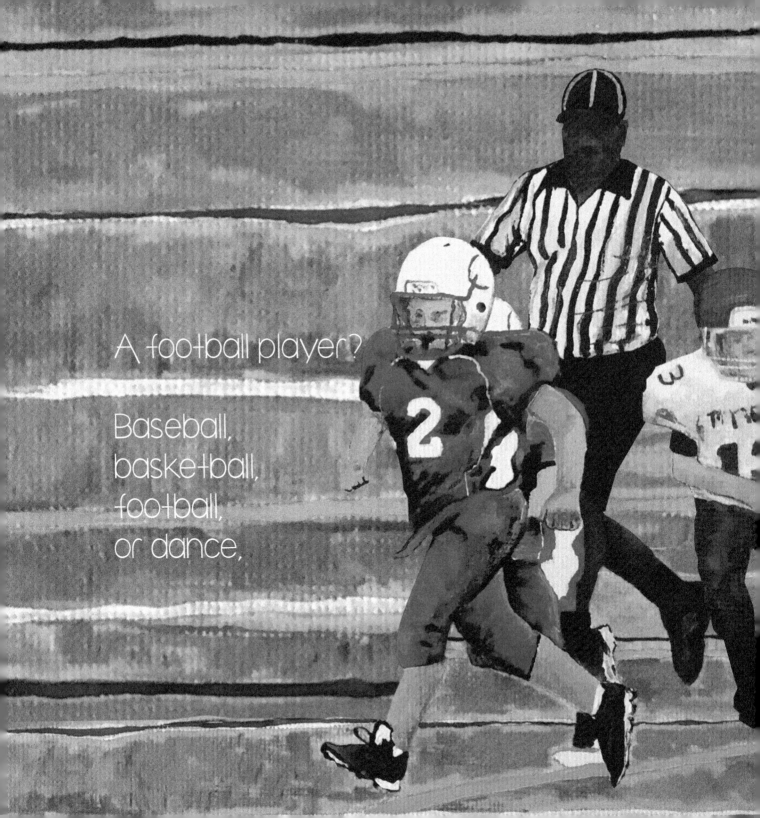

A football player?

Baseball,
basketball,
football,
or dance,

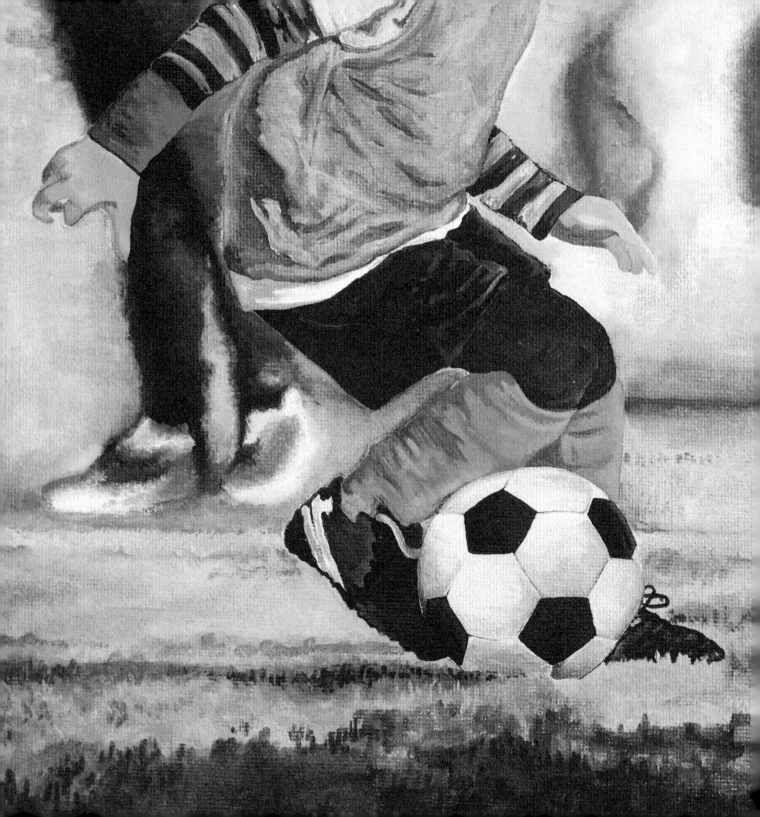

Piano or trumpet
or soccer by chance?

Whatever you love,
whatever cajoles,
eating plants gives you
strength to
achieve all your goals.

Come with me,
I know you'll see,
the pledge is the key
to a healthier life
for you and me.

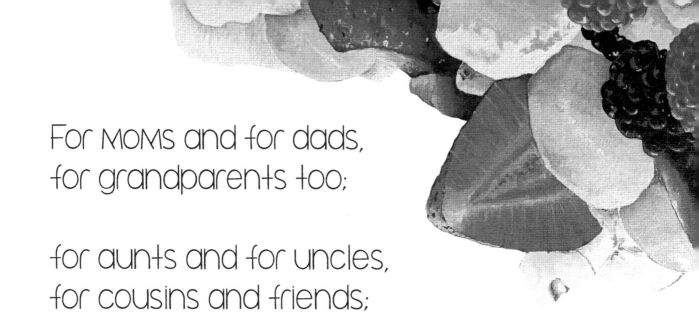

For moms and for dads,
for grandparents too;

for aunts and for uncles,
for cousins and friends;

share it with everyone,
the pledge never ends.

So...what are you waiting for?
Lets begin; plant a garden
together, and
everyone wins!

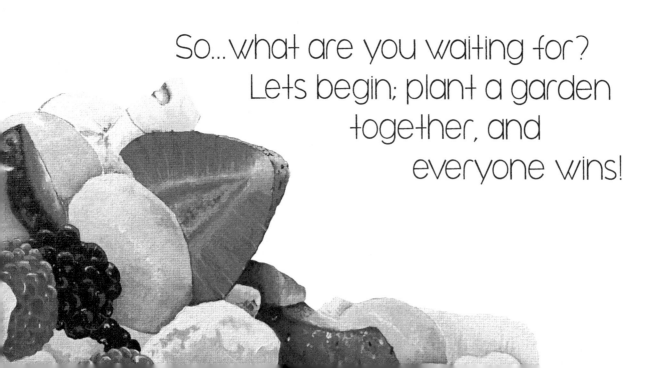

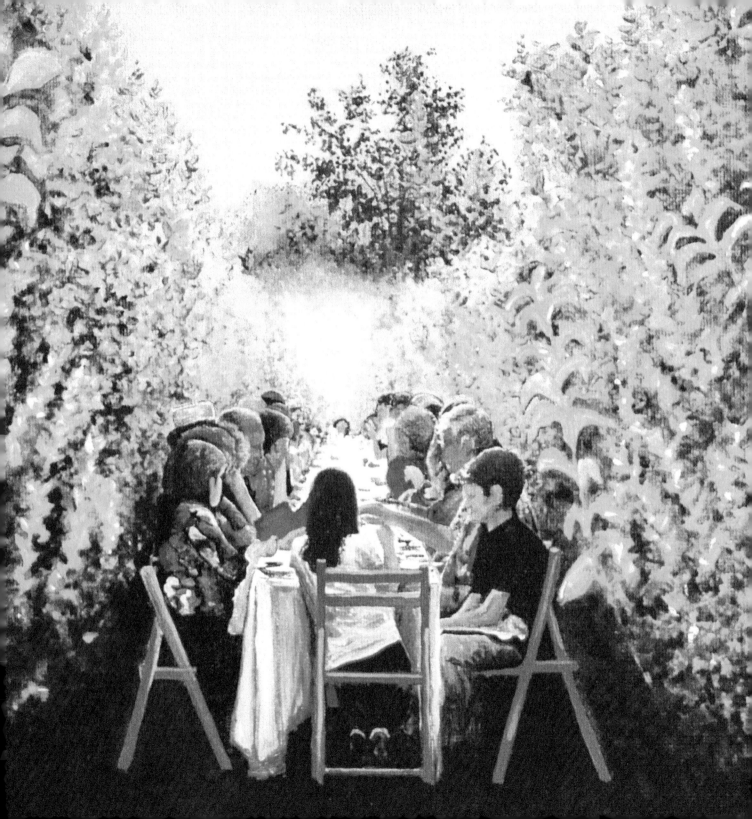

CPSIA information can be obtained
at www.ICGtesting.com
Printed in the USA
BVOW05*2157220517
484892BV00004B/5/P